How to Gain Weight

From Ectomorph to Mesomorph

Khail Kapp

Contents

INTRODUCTION

As she kissed down my neck, collar bone, ribs, disappeared a bit in the canyon that was my abdomen, and took hold of my protruding hip bones... it hits me. I think she could kick my ass. I don't really believe this, but I still allow the thought to cross my mind. I'm embarrassed at how scrawny I look from this angle. I start to notice more and more that it's not necessarily the angle; I'm skin and bones.

Does this sound familiar? Have you been in a situation where you weren't happy with your weight? Are you at a point in life where you would love to gain weight, or been at that point for years? Do you think that you are too tall, too short, too weak or too busy to pack on the pounds? Have you tried everything from counting calories to drinking buckets of weight-gainer? Have you tried supplements, diets, and exercises, and still your metabolism stands victorious above you with a menacing grin? Have you just about given up hope for gaining weight? Don't give up! You are part of a huge community that has found it impossible to gain weight. I have been there and I can tell you how to get out. People that envy your metabolism don't understand that the odds are stacked against you. Yes, it would be easier to gain weight if you were built differently. But, there is hope my friends. There is a way to achieve your goals and build the body you want. There are no secrets here. I will share with you my experiences and insight on how to blow through your metabolism, get stronger, feel more motivated and become more confident. I'll set you on the right path. It will be challenging and it will be fun.

My Story

"Lift is too short to be small." -Timothy Ferriss

Growing up poor meant that food was often scarce. Encouraging me to eat more might have been counterintuitive. I was pretty much raised on mac & cheese and spaghetti, which no child ever complained about. Hindsight is the tough part. I did have a grandmother who seemed concerned with my eating. She would berate me in front of friends and family, humiliating me for being skinny. While visiting, her constant nagging made it impossible for me to eat. But these aren't excuses. I came to find later that it didn't matter what other people thought. I truly did eat like a bird. I was picky and my stomach was the size of a baseball. The thought of finishing my plate made me nauseous. Ordering food from a restaurant gave me anxiety. I knew I needed to eat more, but I didn't want to push through any of that negativity. Put more accurately, I honestly believed that I was incapable. I felt trapped, like I would never be able to change this self-defeating attitude.

Most of my life lessons came through television and anecdotes. I remember believing that a big spaghetti dinner the night before a big game would give me more energy. I later learned that carbs burn fast and mine were gone before they hit my stomach. I remember thinking that big guys ate a lot of hearty meals. I learned later that some of the most buff guys eat a ton of fat and significantly less protein. I thought a balanced diet required helpings of carbs, multiple vegetables, and lots of fruits. This is also a common misconception.

Being a skinny guy took its toll on my confidence. I'd over analyze myself and the clothes that I'd try while looking in the mirror. I'd buy preppy button ups and then never wear them because they just didn't seem to fit me right. While sitting, I'd over bend my knees, tucking my feet under my chair to give the illusion that my legs were thicker. I was never comfortable in my own skin. I was a little obsessed to say the least.

1

When it came to eating, my memories are of nausea. I found it impossible to finish my food most of the time. I would reach a certain point, typically 3/4 of my plate, and my stomach would scream "HALT!" in the ancient language of Feeling Like I Was Going to Hurl. I'd gag, and at times I would even puke. I'd get anxious eating in front of people. Watching my friends easily devour twice my portion was so defeating. I think about these times now like I'm looking back on the very first steps I took. In the tough moments of life where you are trying to break through challenges, the tasks are daunting and you may not even recognize the light at the end of the tunnel. But, I can assure you there is plenty of light and the tunnel is not as deep as you think.

I struggled with putting on weight throughout high school. Even bad weight. I'd eat junior bacon cheeseburgers after workout sessions for protein, and never lost sight of my six-pack. My wrists measured 5" tops. I was 85lbs my freshman year. My metabolism was invincible. When we started conditioning for freshman football I was immensely humbled by the bench press. It took me weeks just to lift the bar (45lbs). This humility didn't last long as I always believed myself to be tough and strong. I was tenacious if anything. I think everyone needs to have a slightly over-confident view of themselves, or at least have a view of their potential. Fixating on your potential can be the driving force you need to keep pushing. We all have a little spark inside, some of us just forget how to wield it.

I was the smallest guy on the team, but what I lacked in size (and skill) I made up for with my big hard head. Staying out of the views of the opposing team, I struck low and hard. I'd rock my head with every tackle. It was decently effective at slowing or bringing down a bigger guy, yet very effective at providing me with multiple concussions. I was also put on special teams as it was quite comical for the coaches to watch my 85lb body get tossed five or six yards.

It was pouring rain. The lights glistened through the raindrops and shimmered off the silver and red helmets of the opposing team. I remember thinking that these guys looked more like a varsity squad from a movie than a freshman football team. The first play of the game I was on kickoff. I never was aware enough to know that I

2

looked like a delicious steak meal to these guys. Or maybe better put, more like a lean little chicken nugget. I only thought about the game and what it would be like to hit the returner so hard that he fumbled. We kicked the ball and I made it about ten yards before I tasted mud. I was rocked so hard from a blind-spot that I flew a few feet and slid across the field. It took me a few minutes to get back up. I felt like it was a cheap move and that it wasn't fair. But the only unfair treatment was the way I was treating my own body. Had I known better ways to take care of myself, had I understood some key principles on weight-gain, I would've been able to take that hit better and even safely land a few more of my own.

Sports would continue to punish my body, giving it the foundation but not all the ingredients it needed to grow muscles. Wrestling wound up being an excellent fit for my size, but anyone who knows anything about wrestling can tell you that it is not the sport where you *put on weight*. It taught me the value of hard work and consistency. I mean, it *drilled* those values into my head. I started out horrible and through two years of rigorous training, wound up being pretty *meh*. Toward the end of my senior career I came down with mono and was bedridden for a week. I spent the days sleeping, and when I wasn't asleep, I was gorging on food. The state of being as relaxed as a cat, snoozing for hours and hours, had calmed my body incredibly. It also built my appetite up quite a bit. I gained 10lbs that week and when the sickness lifted, I felt better than ever. And I was. I finished my wrestling career at the 135-weight class. I ate whatever I wanted, weighed under 132lbs and never wrestled better in my life. What happened? I had a lesson in front of me that I wouldn't learn for another few months.

I am a huge supporter of organized sports, but they don't give you everything you need to bulk. You may already know this if you've been in sports and are asking yourself the same questions. When I graduated high school, organized sports were mostly a thing of the past. Lifting would be my new sport and I was determined to finally have the body I desired.

I commuted to a branch campus of Penn State for my freshman year. Moving in with my dad, I'd save a few grand driving to school. My dad is a big guy. He's built like a big guy and so it goes with his side of the family. My mother's side is the exact opposite. My beautiful sisters are built like models, while my bone structure is tiny and lanky. I have long legs, long arms, a shorter torso, a fat neck and a big head. The last two I can thank my dad for. Making my body match my head was a decent goal to strive for, one that would require a lot of weight gain in the right places.

My dad also ate like a big guy. The fridge was always stocked with chicken, steaks, bacon, eggs, and deli meats and cheeses. And this is where the right kind of weight gain started. He would grill every night, always more food than we needed. We would eat dinner in front of James Bond marathons until I was stuffed. He would clean up and tell me to pick at the leftovers on my plate for a while. He encouraged me to eat more with every meal we had together. Before long I was eating a little more food than I was used to. I realized that if I ate until I was nauseous, the nausea would pass, and then I could eat a tiny bit more. I'd get a little nauseous, stop and wait, and then take another bite. Dinner was a good place to practice this as the audience didn't mind my uneasy facial expressions or the fact that it took me over an hour to finish eating. Before long I was eating double!

The small branch campus had a few dorms, three large buildings for classes, and a tiny gym containing most of the basics in quantities of one. My plan was simple: schedule classes with a break every day to hit the gym and eat a good lunch. I made friends with some guys in the dorms, and after most workouts, would crash on their couch for a half hour or so. Other days I'd catch a nap in my car, or front and center of my favorite class. Feeling refreshed upon waking, I'd proceed to eat lunch while taking notes. I had no shame sleeping or eating in front of people because my goal was righteous. I wanted to gain weight and I was willing to do it at any (natural) cost.

I developed a consistent schedule revolving around **eating**, sleeping, and working out. I'd wake up early, pound a protein shake, make bacon and eggs, and head to class. I'd have a snack during class and then hit the gym. After the gym, I'd have a protein shake, a nap, and then lunch. I'd usually get another snack in before dinner, making sure to get to bed at a decent time so I'd get 8 hours, I'd sleep like a baby. Rinse and repeat. In six months, I had put on 30lbs and significantly improved my strength in all aspects. But this fantasy world with time for napping and a personal chef only lasted for a year.

I've since learned much more about dieting, exercising, and maintaining/manipulating mass. I've gained 10lbs of muscle in a month. I've even repeated 30lbs in six months. **I don't expect anyone reading this to have the cushy life I had my freshman year.** I am a realist. I have achieved strength and weight gains while working full time and having a 2 hour commute each way. I've done it while working from 2:00 p.m. to 2:00 a.m. This kind of weight gain can happen in your life even if you work long hours, have long skinny limbs, and think my sentences are long-winded. If you are finally ready to commit to gaining weight, I can show you how to do it. The following will elaborate on the ingredients you need to put on mass, feel more confident in your birthday suit, and avoid trips to the ER every time your hip bumps a table.

MOTIVATION

"They tried to bury us. They didn't know we were seeds." -Dinos
Christianopoulos

Before starting a new habit, before making a serious commitment,
before making nearly any important decision, you must be
motivated. Your motivation is the key to unlocking the potential of
your ideal self and so much more. Hopefully your purchase of this
book means that you've decided that enough was enough, and it's
time to beef up. But just in case, I'd like to elaborate. When I was a
kid, I was motivated by laughter, so I became the class clown. Later,
I was motivated by women, and I was just as successful at making
myself a clown. When your motivation is weak or you are motivated
for the wrong reasons, you are doomed to fail. Eventually, I'd lose
my work ethic, my motivation, and obviously and easily, I'd lose
any of my hard-earned muscle.

All my hard-earned accomplishments in life have had the same key
ingredients. They start with the proper motivation, which requires
self-focus. Why do you want to make a change? What will this
change mean for you and how will it make you feel to experience
this change? Set yourself a goal where you can measure your
progress, remind yourself regularly of the goal, and have a laser
focus on accomplishing that goal. More eating and lifting are things
you can control and measure. Believe me, once you begin to practice
these things regularly, your boost in energy and hormones, your
feeling of overall well-being, and your reflection in the mirror will
boost your confidence. Your confidence will in turn help you to stay
committed. But it won't stop there. Building a solid physical
foundation is a gateway drug to building a mental one. Challenging
yourself regularly is the only true path to success. Fitness has helped
my confidence in work, nearly doubling my annual income year over
year for five years. Money isn't everything in life, although it can
solve a ton of problems. But confidence and learning to love and

trust myself has brought me great friends, a beautiful and wild family, and the admiration and respect of my siblings and parents. This book is focused on gaining weight, but I believe you will gain more than that.

I am a firm believer in empowering people. My opinion: if you don't do this for yourself, above everyone else, you won't stay fully committed. That's not to say that you shouldn't use your spouse, your kids, your friends or your crush as motivators. But you need to put yourself in front of them at some point. It's kind of like fixating your oxygen mask before you apply your child's. If you can't be content/happy/confident with yourself, you're doing your loved ones a disservice. They will appreciate you more when you are happy and satisfied with yourself, which will make them happier. People will like being around you more when you are happier with yourself, which in turn will lead to more successful interactions. Maybe your confidence is not an issue. I still believe that having a better body will make your life better and happier. You've been frustrated that putting weight on has been challenging - to say the least? Let's see if we can remove that stressor from your life once and for all.

Write down your thoughts, your concerns, your difficulties and your aggravations. Try to think of specific times that have sat with you. Try to feel how you've felt. Ask yourself what this is costing you. Is it costing you your happiness? Your confidence? How much time do you spend thinking about your body? How often? Couldn't you be thinking about something more positive or productive? Write your thoughts below. Seriously. Just write something. Anything. It seems silly but it is important!

Now visualize your ideal self. Write down a weight you would like to be, an arm circumference you would like to have, or a shirt size you would like to fit in. You decide what you would like to focus on. Imagine how different you will feel as you get closer to this goal. That positivity, that visualization will be your driver.

———————————————————————————

———————————————————————————

———————————————————————————

I am a big believer in being mindful of the things I tell myself on a regular basis. This is pertinent to having a positive attitude. Staying positive makes committing to new habits much easier. If you've accomplished a great feat in the past, something that made you proud, how did you get there? How did it make you feel? Know that you're committed to this for a good reason. If you feel like this situation is hopeless, or like there is no way to force rapid and positive change in your life, you're wrong! But, you aren't alone by any means. If you believe you can't gain weight or strength no matter what you do, I hear you. You need to understand that you are capable of nearly anything when you're focused on yourself and committed. If you haven't heard about the good wolf and the bad wolf, I'm going to describe this concept below. If you have, read it anyway!

Inside of you there are two wolves. The good wolf motivates and empowers you. The good wolf takes you forward through life, helping you grow and learn. The bad wolf drags you down, wants to keep you in bed in the morning, wants you to seek approval from your peers through negative behaviors, and encourages you to put effort and energy into trivial things in your life. The bad wolf makes you think you are incapable. At the end of this wolf story, the wolves will fight, and the wolf you feed the most will win. **Which wolf are you feeding more?** Everything we do, everyone we associate with, and everything we watch and listen to, is food for the wolves. Ask yourself frequently: How is my attitude? How are the attitudes of those around me, and how is this making me feel? Ask yourself if what you are doing right now is going to build you up? If it isn't, maybe it is time to reconsider some of your daily activities. When you decide to stay up an extra few hours to watch TV, and then sleep in and miss the gym, was it worth it? Every time you allow yourself to believe you can't gain weight or get stronger, you are feeding that bad wolf. Try to take note of how many minutes or even hours you spend a day on social media for practice. You aren't going to wake up one day and be surprised at your weight gain. Instead, you are going to watch yourself progressively grow, while consistently telling yourself you are capable.

Work the body and the mind will thank you. If you feel negatively about your weight or just generally about yourself, trust me, exercise can have tremendous effects on your psyche. If you're already an avid exerciser, great! You are here to gain weight and now that you are committed, let's get to it.

EAT MORE

"Whether you think you can, or you think you can't — either way you're right." -Henry Ford

Eating more always sounds easier than it is. You will watch people eat as if eating was their sport. You may believe they are designed differently than you. You may believe you have pushed your limits to their max when it comes to eating. The thing about over-eating that makes it so difficult is the combination between physical pain and mental distress. The physical part manifests itself as tension, uneasiness, and nausea. The mind begins to stress, which leads to doubt. Worst of all you may tell yourself, "If it feels this way, it must be wrong!" I'm going to give you the bad news right off the bat. When it comes to any type of fitness, whether it's gaining or losing weight, getting ripped or jacked or even sumo, dieting is about 80% of the battle. Some find the dieting to be the hardest part. Some make it overly confusing by counting calories and measuring their every activity. In reality, just forcing yourself to overeat is all you need. Dieting is simply just another factor to control. We are all capable of adjusting our diets (within our financial means), and I will provide the insight you need to begin adjusting yours.

Do a quick Wiki search for Matt "Megatoad" Stonie. This guy weighs a whopping 120lbs at 5'8", yet holds several titles for eating contests. I'm always fascinated with champion eaters and their ability to eat so much and so quickly. Their ability is almost super-human. *Almost*. What is their secret? **Stomach Expansion.** The stomach is an amazing organ. It is made up of 3 layers of muscle, it secretes acid strong enough to eat through wood (don't try this at home), and is plastic. Plasticity means it can change physical shape. A typical example used is the over-stuffing of everyone's bellies on Thanksgiving. I prefer to think about all those failed stomach staple surgeries. Bypassing most of the stomach's space allows a patient to feel full quicker. In reality, the problem could often solve itself with a little more willpower. Patients whom this surgery fails usually wind up stretching the remaining usable portion of the stomach into the size of the original stomach. The stomach is capable of some insane stretching! How fortunate for us. A human stomach can often fit over a gallon of material. How close do you think your average meal gets you to a gallon?

Stomach expansion requires relaxation. Part of the secret behind those world record eaters is the speed at which they eat. But that isn't the most important part. If you eat faster, you don't give your body enough time to start the digestion process. Therefore, you can fill up your stomach before it starts contracting. I was never a fast eater and wouldn't claim to be one today. Initially, what you need is enough time and just like with me, dinner is a great place to start. When you sit down to your next meal, focus only on eating. Eat as quickly as you can without looking like a crazy person or making yourself throw up. Chew thoroughly as well. This sounds elementary but your soon-to-be over-stuffed stomach will be thankful it has less work to do. As you slow down, just keep drudging forward. Wait until you couldn't possibly eat another bite. Wait a few minutes, and do just that. Eat another bite or eat what you can. Continue this cycle until you run out of time, but don't hurt yourself. Just know that your stomach has a lot of room, so stretch it out a little bit! Remind yourself that you can make room. Remind yourself that you are eating for the sole purpose of gaining weight. Start eating more often and make all your meals into a gorging experience. Save your drinks for the end of the meal or try to sip. There is always room for water, but food real-estate is hard to come by. Your nausea and tight stomach will be things of the past. You just need to desensitize this reflex of getting nauseous or full too quickly. With the right attitude, you can accelerate this process!

Here's the most common theme I will try to impart to you: be consistent. If you overeat for a few days and then decide to eat light, your stomach will shrink. Think about it this way: you have X number of years being skinny vs. Y number of days/months you've been overeating. Your body is going to want to return to its original state. Keep up with the overeating. Every day you will be able to eat a little bit more each meal.

Keeping a Log
Many bodybuilders weigh out all their food servings, measuring protein and other nutrient intake down to the gram. If you decide to use a scale, purchase a decent one. We do need to make sure you are eating a little bit more every day. An easy tool to use is a measuring cup, and just do a quick Google search on what the nutritional value is if you're keeping track of protein. Be sure to measure once your food is fully prepared to ensure accuracy. You can also keep a log of meals every day on a spreadsheet or easy to access file. The MyFitnessPal App is a great and free resource you can use to get a good idea of how many calories you are getting for each food item you're eating. I recommend downloading something like this to stay organized and get a good understanding of what you need to be eating. But I would advise not just using the app, but focusing more on how you are eating and continually pushing yourself. Make sure you log your meals right away so that you don't lose track or inadvertently input false data. Be sure to always push yourself to eat a little bit more than the last time you ate that meal, even if it is just a bite. Keeping a log will demonstrate progress, which will be an important confidence booster when you feel any doubt. If you miss an opportunity to log information, just keep yourself honest and make sure you are applying stomach expansion with every meal! It will become second nature very quickly!

But I Really Can't Eat Another Bite!
Not with that attitude! I love to say this comment at inappropriate or ironic times. (Wife: "Khail, I can't possibly miss another day of work!" Khail: "Not with that attitude.") In this case, I really mean it. Your attitude is the conversation you have with yourself. You can either be your biggest supporter or your worst nightmare. What do you want? To build your body into an ideal shape? Or to have a comfy life where you don't push yourself, feeling incapable or like a victim? Know that pushing yourself to achieve what you want is incredibly rewarding. This applies not just to your body, but to all

aspects of life. People become happier, better sleepers, better lovers, more confident, and even more financially successful when they trust themselves. All trust is earned. Set a goal and work toward accomplishing it. I was scrawny and there's a good chance I was smaller than you with my bone structure. Just know that you aren't alone in having a crazy metabolism and that your stomach is not different. It just needs to be desensitized through practice. Plus, you will be able to wield that metabolism later to get sexier results and your hardships could turn out to be gifts in disguise!

What to Eat
I've counted calories. I've set the bar high to try to get fast results and failed miserably. The apps work great and counting calories is a proven way to manipulate weight. It works especially well when losing or maintaining weight. However, I believe in quality over quantity when it comes to gaining the right kind of weight. If you're only interested in packing on weight period, hear me out. Your metabolism might be able to handle entire chocolate cakes for 3 meals a day, but you won't have the energy or the protein to build muscle with that. Ask yourself, is this food going to help build my body or is it simply satisfying my mood? Certainly, enjoy your food and put effort into your meals so that you can look forward to stuffing yourself. But, people often get caught up in treating eating like something more than it is. You may find sooner or later that it doesn't matter what it tastes like if it works and it is giving you fuel.

You want to focus heavily on **protein** intake. Bulking usually means at least getting 1 gram of protein per pound of current body weight. I've eaten much more and too much protein can be a waste. Not enough protein and you will be sore longer and won't see any gain in mass. Try to find you're sweet-spot! If you are picky, it is time to start trying different things. Just one more behavior you can and will get used to. Tuna and other fish are excellent sources of lean protein, but be mindful that larger fish contain high levels of mercury, so limit your intake as there can be side-effects. Other great sources of protein include chicken, eggs, beef, jerky (get a food dehydrator!), nuts, bone broth, peanut or almond butter, tahini, and protein supplements. My favorite type of supplements include

Hydrolyzed Whey and Casein from Optimum Nutrition and Gatorade Protein Bars. If shakes make you as queasy as they made me: try finding a flavor you like, try mixing it with just water to make it thinner, choose hydrolyzed because it mixes like chocolate milk, or add a little salt! What you want to make sure you do is remain consistent. Keep trying to desensitize your uneasiness. Greek yogurt might take a little, and I mean a very little, getting used to. But, it is a fantastic source of protein and great for digestion. You will want to take care of your system while you are punishing it. Avoid soy-based products by checking your protein sources under ingredients. ***But Khail, I don't eat meat or anything of the sort!*** Lucky for you, the world is full of healthy and protein-filled treats. Beans, lentils, and quinoa are great and tasty sources of protein. I ate a strict diet with lentils and beans and packed on significant muscle while burning fat in just a month! If your weight doesn't increase after a week of honest overeating, try increasing your protein intake or adding another set to each exercise.

Myth: Fat is bad for you. The reality is that sugar and most carbs are bad for you. The right amount of fat is good for you if you are getting your fat from the right places. You can effectively lose weight eating a high fat, moderate protein diet just by cutting out the sugars and most of the carbs. Good fats come from walnuts, almonds, cashews and other nuts. Olive oil, coconut oil, and even butter and cheese are good sources as well. Avocado is a fantastic source too! I like dipping chicken in guacamole to avoid the empty carbs and to make people uncomfortable around me. The old-school thought was to avoid fat at all costs.

Next, to fight the almost inevitable, constant trips to the toilet throughout the day you need to increase your **fiber**. Get used to eating salads, spinach, asparagus, broccoli, kale, and other leafy veggies. Without these, you're sure to waste much of that protein you are struggling to fit into your stomach. I would often take 4-5 trips to the bathroom a day and continue to struggle gaining weight until I increased my fiber intake. Throw kale in a skillet for a few minutes with some olive oil and dry garlic. Cooked kale tastes much better than the raw stuff and I prefer the opposite for baby spinach. Honestly, I eat a handful or two of baby spinach raw from the bag every morning with my hard-boiled eggs and leftover bacon (usually standing over the trashcan so I don't have to use a plate).

If you're trying to put on only good weight, limit your **fruit** intake as it is mostly sugar. If you're worried about vitamins, take some supplements. Don't reach for fruit juice unless it's when you are boozing. Juice is a much better choice than soda. And as much as you aren't going to want to hear this depending on your age, alcohol is sugar too. Overall, the effects of drinking on your physique are tremendous. If you can limit yourself and cut out drinking completely. People can lose a ton of unwanted weight when they stop drinking, and skinny folks can put on weight (especially muscle) easier when sober. If you're a regular soda drinker, cut it out. I've only known one person that could drink copious amounts of soda and keep a stellar physique. Obviously candy and sweets aren't going to build muscle, so cut them out as often as possible. If you're problem is not eating enough, you are wasting space in your belly with dessert. For dessert, have another meal! No joke. Reach for protein instead of ice cream at night.

Drink milk and eat cheese if you can. They even make lactose-free stuff now. These are great fat and protein sources. When I was packing on the pounds, buffalo chicken pizza with a milk-based protein shake were typical lunches. I usually avoid carbs and gluten now, but with moderation, these will give you quick energy and won't put on bad weight. Given your metabolism, you may even find that cutting carbs is irrelevant to maintain low bodyfat. Just keep in mind what you are filling your belly with. A huge, bready hoagie is taking up real estate for protein, fat and fiber.

When to Eat
Always. Eat as often as you can and be sure to eat breakfast. Eating breakfast and grazing frequently will boost your metabolism, giving you the ability to eat more but also speeding up the way your body processes this stuff. You will find that you have more room earlier in the day. **But I can't wake up!** I was like you, and I am still not a morning person. Try cooking yourself a delicious breakfast every morning. You may not want to roll out of bed- but bacon! I am a good arguer.

It is common knowledge that eating late at night leads to weight gain. SO, eat at night. Try to get 5-6 meals in per day but ultimately make sure you are eating enough protein. **Pack a lunch** to make sure you have enough. If you work odd hours, always over pack so that you're prepared. If you have a long commute, use that time (safely), eat! Have a protein bar in the car, stash a snack in the work bathroom, empty your filing cabinets and fill your folders with pancakes. You get the idea. Another important point, focus on yourself. Others aren't going to understand why you're eating like this. The mesomorph across the table is going to brag about how lean his lunch is, but you are different. You haven't been able to gain weight in the past, and now you're going to.

Eating all day may provide enough calories but may not effectively stretch your stomach. You may only be filling your stomach all day long. This was the problem I had with counting calories and why I couldn't see gains. Stomach expansion with every meal! Below is what a typical day looked like by the time I had gained 30lbs, so if it seems like too much, it might be. It took time in the gym and practicing over-stuffing myself to get to this point. You can tweak it to your specifications.

Sample Weight Gaining Meal Plan:

Wake-up: Protein shake with milk within twenty minutes of waking up. Hearty breakfast: several pieces of bacon, 4-6 eggs with spinach cooked in, peanut butter toast (something crunchy always helps me eat more). I've also been known to put mixed veggies and broccoli in my eggs.

Don't cook mixed greens or lettuce in eggs as these get oily/watery and make that omelet into something nasty.

Snack: Trail mix with cashews, walnuts, dried cranberries and dark chocolate. Beef jerky or protein bar, etc. Throw in some fiber like a handful of baby spinach.

Post-Gym Protein Shake

Lunch: Chicken breasts, or a stacked deli-meat sandwich/wrap, tuna, steak, burger, or anything else along those lines will work. When choosing sides, try a salad. Chips and candy aren't your friends anymore. If this isn't enough by this time of day, switch to eating two lunches before and after the time you would normally eat lunch.

Snack: Same as before

Dinner: Big and hearty as often as possible with a focus on protein. If you're going to have pasta, make sure you're stocking up on the meatballs. I like a traditional meat, potatoes and green vegetable meal. Sweet potatoes are fantastic as well.

Snack: Same as above, or eat your leftovers.

Pre-Bed: Casein Protein with milk.

Throughout the day, drink a ton of water. I always carry a stainless-steel water bottle and fill it constantly. I keep a gallon jug in my car so I won't run out of water on long commutes. I find that most minor ailments can be treated by drinking water, especially headaches. Without enough water, you're not going to get the results you're about to work so hard for. I typically drink 4-6 20oz bottles a day.

To maintain this gain, be consistent. I eat the same thing nearly every day. This saves on money, brain power and prep time, and in turn you will have more time to focus on other important aspects of your life. It ensures that I always have the amount of food I need on hand, so I don't walk into work trying to calculate protein content from a Chinese food menu. I do meal prep on Sundays. I grill enough chicken all at once to feed myself for the next week or so. I have glass storage containers that keep foods fresh longer. If you have space for it, start a small garden for kale and spinach. Buying a few containers and cooking all your meals for the week or even the month can be a huge game changer for your health and weight gain. This stuff seems excessive but it is merely practical.

As you push yourself in the gym, your appetite will improve tremendously. While you're eating, remind yourself that you are eating for fuel. Remember that your stomach can and will expand. When you decide that you are eating your last bite, really scrutinize yourself. Can you fit more? Know that you are on a mission to gain weight and nothing is going to stop you now.

WORKING OUT

"Strength does not come from winning. Your struggles develop your strengths. When you go through hardships and decide not to surrender, that is strength." -Arnold Schwarzenegger

Whether you are brand new to the gym or you have plateaued, looking at the gym from a fresh lens will be important. Although diet may be upwards of 80% of the problem when it comes to acquiring the physique of your dreams, there will be no good gains without hard work. There are an infinite number of routines and theories that may work for you. I've tried and been successful with many, and I've documented some great examples at the end of this chapter. Not everything will fit your lifestyle. I've had such varying lifestyles over the years that one of my routines is bound to be a good match for you. You may only be able to spare half an hour a week, or you may find that you have more time than you think. Being honest with yourself is of ultimate importance when trying to accomplish any difficult goal. Take note of how often you are spending time on things that aren't helping you achieve your goals. If you are addicted to social media, TV, the night life, or whatever you do behind closed doors, ask yourself how these things are helping you pack on muscle. You might find that you can free up an extra hour or more every day simply by cutting back or eliminating just one of these vices.

Finding What Works

There are essential principles that must be understood before going forward. Hopefully, some of these are new to you. If you know these already, the dieting may be the only ingredient you've been lacking. Either way, I'd encourage you to really dig into the details here and BE HONEST.

It is Not *How Much* You Lift, but *How* You Lift
Form over everything. If you can curl 50lb dumbbells but you're rocking like you're drunk at 3:00 a.m. on an old ship in a storm, you can't curl 50lb dumbbells. Trust me, your results from curling 20lb dumbbells with a steady back will be much better than doing 'the sway'. If the exercise is for your biceps, make sure your biceps are doing all the work. If you're benching, keep that butt on the bench. There are plenty of exercises that focus on multiple muscle groups, but the theme here is to make sure you are only working those groups.

Everybody started somewhere. Don't focus on the number. Eventually it will be a number you are proud of, but until then, be proud of the fact that you are in there doing the hard work. Be proud you are focused on the result. The weight doesn't matter. You are doing this for you, so ignore the guy next to you. If you must look, take notes on form or use the perfect physical specimen as motivation. If you want the quick-fix and think a shortcut is your answer, I would challenge that. The reward you will feel from the hard work you put in to naturally develop those muscles will be far greater than what you would receive from using steroids. Have pride, have confidence, and have fun working hard.

Another very important part of good form is preservation. Your future self will thank you for focusing on form. If you're not concerned with that person right now, know that you need to avoid injury to get the gains you're looking for. Focus on form. Take your time. Be honest. Push yourself correctly. There is no point in lifting heavy weight if it means you're cheating. These are your essentials. If you have the humility, ask someone at the gym for advice. A little tweak could mean the world. If you're not up for face-to-face criticism, there are millions of resources for body building and proper form online.

My Favorite Pearls and Terms
Squats: Pick a place above and in front of you to stare at. Keep your eyes focused on that spot throughout the rep. It will help you

to keep your chin up, which helps to keep your back straight and to prevent injuries and falling forward. Do your best to give your legs the full range of motion by bending them to 90°. Remember, quality over quantity!

Don't Bounce: Don't bounce the bar off your chest. Don't bounce the weights off the floor. The bounce is cheating and isn't making you stronger. I bounced the bar off my chest until I cracked my sternum and the weird thing still pops like a knuckle when I stretch.

Squeeze: At the end of the rep, squeeze the muscle. As your muscles get bigger, this becomes easier to do. A great example can be felt in calve raises. Squeeze and hold your flexed calve at the top of the rep before slowly going back to rest.

Playlist: I either choose from a few good Pandora stations, or a personalized playlist that gets me in the mood to toss around some iron. Music is a great motivator, but feel free to listen to NPR if you would rather add culture to your crunch-session.

Negatives: When you are returning the weights to a neutral position (i.e. when the bar is being lowered to your chest in bench), go slowly. You can push slowly or you can explode, both have benefits, but it is important to be very controlled when returning to a neutral position. You can make an entire exercise significantly harder by concentrating on form and going as slow as possible.

Failure: A failure is when you give it everything you've got until your muscles give out. Completing your sets with failures is an excellent way to gain strength and size, and ultimately to break through walls. Be sure to ask for a spotter for these sets when doing anything that you can't safely drop.

Super-Set: Instead of taking a break in between sets, pick an opposing muscle group to work. Examples include bouncing back and forth from a chest to a back routine, biceps to triceps, or something unrelated like shoulders or abs with legs. If you have the energy, this method screams efficiency!

Ending on a Good Note: It is important to leave the gym every day feeling accomplished. Do your favorite exercises last and you will leave with more positive feelings, which will motivate you to return. If there are exercises you dislike or you are unable to put up much weight on, start with these. Get them over with first. I believe Mark Twain's frog eating example works well here.

Mix it Up: Don't do the same workouts for the rest of your life. Find new ways to target your muscle groups. Put emphasis on this pearl if you aren't getting any bigger or stronger. I try to change up my routine every two months or so, but I know successful guys who try something different every session. However, we want to measure our results, so stay consistent until you hit a wall.

Don't Avoid Abs: Don't neglect any muscle group for that matter, but I choose abs specifically because as a skinny guy, I always felt like I didn't need to work my abs. Your core needs to grow in strength with the rest of you, or you're sure to get injured.

Routine

Should I go to the gym in the morning or at night? The answer to this question is very simple. <u>Go when you will.</u> You need to make sure you consistently go to the gym or it will all be for nothing. If it is hard for you to get your finger off the snooze button, the morning may not be for you. But if your life doesn't allot for a good chunk of time to yourself, you may want to reconsider. I lift first thing in the morning because it is a time I know that I can go. After a long day of work, the last thing I want to do is hit the gym. The to-do list always manages to grow as the day goes on. I wasn't a morning person at all until I started cooking breakfast for myself and going to the gym. When I worked 12 hour days, the morning was the only time I could commit to. When I had a long commute, after work was the perfect time to wind down and get some 'me time'. I had to pass the gym on my way home anyway, so it was only practical to stop in and get my swell on. If you have a family or other similar commitments, I'd say get in the habit of working out in the morning. Unless you think you can break away after the kids go to sleep? Ultimately, I recommend choosing the time that is the hardest for you to skip. We are trying to build a habit here, which requires consistency. Pick a time and stick to it!

Can't Go to the Gym? If you are absolutely sure there is no time in your life to go to the gym, not a single hour to spare a week, I don't believe you. But I'll try to help you find ways to work out either way. Get a yoga mat. If you can't afford one, use an old towel or draw a big rectangle on your carpet with magic marker. Put it in a place where it can lay constantly. Lay it next to your bed if need be. In the morning, stretch, and do as many push-ups, sit-ups, and squats as you can. If you have time, do multiple sets. Repeat the exercises at night and remember to push yourself. In the shower, flex your muscles. Push your palms together in front of your chest, squeezing your pecs. Get a grip-strengthener for the car ride. Squeeze your abs while sitting. Invest in a pull-up bar or find a place to do them. How often can you work a few muscles while at work? Can you do some exercise related squats in the bathroom? Take the stairs. Ride a bike. Walk your pets. Walk your kids. Carry your spouse. You get the picture. If you are committed, you will invent ways to challenge your muscles. Later in this chapter, I will describe how to pack on muscle with about an hour per week in the gym.

How Often Should I Gym? I love this question as I've experimented quite a bit with this. When it was harder to gain weight, I felt like 2 days away from the gym was detrimental to my gain. I never felt sore on Sundays, so I was effectively skipping a day that I could've been working out. I switched to going 6 days a week. Now, I work out 3-4 days in a row, and then have a rest day or two in between. I also don't like looking at my biological clock as a 7-day week. If we didn't have jobs, the day of the week would almost always be irrelevant. **If you have the energy and you aren't sore in the specific area you are trying to work, go to the gym.** On your rest days, it is still good to get some form of exercise. Maybe make this a cardio or yoga day. Cardio for burning calories and cutting weight is not your aim. But, keeping up your stamina and building your energy levels can be achieved through a half hour or so of cardio per week without sacrificing weight gain. I will include sample plans later that can tweak for your schedule.

How Long Should I Gym? This is another great question. It depends on how sore you are the next day or two afterwards. If you are sore for two days after your workout, I'd say that you are pushing yourself well. When I was younger, I was never sore for more than a day. Then again, I didn't push myself nearly as hard as I do now. You can maximize a twenty-minute gym session by super-setting. If you have time, I'd say the longer you work out, the more your appetite will increase and the easier you'll gain. More time at the gym means you can take longer breaks and lift heavier, or you can squeeze other muscle groups into your routine and lower the number of days in a row you attend. Just judge it off soreness. If you stay at the gym for 2 hours just to talk, your sore jaw muscles won't be enough to increase your appetite. Remember why you're there. Push yourself to make yourself proud, and have fun.

How many sets should I do? How many reps? Everyone will claim to have their own secret formula for size. The general truth is that higher reps and lighter weight equals cut and not size. Another general rule is lifting heavy weight with low reps builds strength and size. I like to do a good combination between the two. Just know that you are different than the guy next to you, and you may need to experiment with what works for you. Again, monitoring your soreness. The first thing you need to do is **keep a log**. There are apps, you can carry a notepad, but whatever you do, just make sure you do it consistently. I use my calendar app to keep track of what and when because it is easy to reference. The title will be the muscle group (i.e. Legs) and the notes will have specific exercises, the setting I adjusted the equipment to, the weights used and number of reps, and any other notes that might be helpful for reference (i.e. I was weak today because I slept poorly). This is incredibly helpful at times, very simple and easy to keep track of. I look back at the last day I worked a specific muscle and I get a good idea of which where to start. As in, if I'm wondering what to do for triceps and last week I ended skull crushers on 110lbs and started on 40lbs, I think it would be safe to start on 50lbs this week. I can search for the muscle group or the specific exercise. As for reps and sets, I mix it up every day in the gym. Not doing the same exact routine every time is great for 'shocking the body' and continuing to develop instead of hitting walls, but not always the best for measuring results. At the very least, I wouldn't recommend the same routine more than two or three months in a row.

Some of My Favorite Examples of Sets/Reps:

Pyramids: These require a spotter or that you're using a machine instead of free weights. Start with whatever weight you can do 10-

12 times before failing. Add weight (i.e. 10lbs) and do 8-10 reps, then 6-8, 4-6, until you're at 2 reps (adding weight each time). The last 2-3 reps are your failure. You can go down to one rep if you think you can get a single rep without cheating.

Drop Sets: Start heavy and work your way to light. Start with something you can't rep more than 5 times, drop the weight by 20-25% and do as many reps as possible, dropping the weight again and again. Get at least 4 sets or until you start doing less reps even as you lower the weight.

Resistance: Example: Slide a bench into the squat rack and set the safety bars just above your chest (so that the barbell can't crush you). Add another 20 or so pounds to your max on the bar. Have a partner help you lift it. Using the squat rack to glide the barbell down, as controlled and slowly as possible, lower the barbell to the safety bars just above your chest. Repeat these a few times at the end of your chest routine and prepare for chest agony for a few days. Negative resistance routines are my number one cure for breaking through plateau periods.

4x5: Heavy weight, do 4 sets of 5 reps. Tweak this to your liking. Try 10 sets of 5.

3x8: I do a lot of 3-5 sets of 8-10 reps. These are good routines when you don't have a partner as you typically won't need a spotter until your last reps.

Burnouts: These are best reserved for the end of your routine. Using significantly less weight than your max, do as many reps as you possibly can! Just in case this is too vague, pick a weight you can do 10-20 times instead of 176 times.

21's: While standing, take a curl bar/EZ-bar/straight-bar, and curl it to 90°. Stop and let it back down. Repeat 7 times. Complete the 7th lower-half curl all the way up to your chest, lower the bar so that your arms are again at 90°, stop and lift back to chest level. Complete 7 of these upper-half curls, straighten your arms down, and complete 7 agonizing full curls. The weight should be enough so that you're crying by the end, but you can at least get close to completing the routine. Similar routines can be done with triceps and leg curls.

Crazy-8's: Start with a weight you can curl 10-12 times. Curl 8, pass to a partner to curl 8, then curl 7 times. Repeat this down to 1 rep and then back up to 8, breaking only to allow your partner to work.

What if it isn't working?
If you're stuck at the same level of strength for a month and you've rules out sleeping or eating more, you need change. Change the set-to-rep ratio or the style (3x8 vs. drop sets). Change the muscle groups you work together, focus more heavily on the thing that is stuck, try slowing down or adding an explosive pull/push to your rep, or take 1-2 weeks off! That last one sounds crazy, but you would be astonished at how well this works. If you've been an active lifter for some time, this might be the first place to start. I try to take 2-4 weeks off per year to ensure I am getting the right amount of rest. Don't think that there is something supernatural holding you back, rather try to get creative with your routine and reassess.

No More Excuses
Do whatever it takes to keep yourself consistent. Remember to ask yourself what you value more. Do I value building the physique I want over grabbing beers with friends? Do I value rolling back and forth under the covers for another 45 minutes in the morning over doing something I can be proud of? There are ways to keep you yourself honest and on the right track. Using friends or partners as motivators can help. Make a bet with someone to keep your commitment on track. Have a silly punishment that deters you from skipping like a 'swear jar' or something similar. Some people are highly motivated by these outside factors. I personally need to look myself in the mirror and have a little chat sometimes. How much energy/time/heart are you willing to put into gaining weight? Ask yourself this question again. If the answer is 'whatever it takes,' you will succeed.

Should I Lift with a Partner?
If you need to find one first, then no. Get to the gym now. If you have one already, keep a few things in mind. Does this person continue to motivate you and refrain from finding excuses for not going to the gym? Are they following a similar fitness path? Someone that is less experienced may give you confidence and

more purpose, but may also be more prone to skipping. Someone who is more experienced may keep you in check more often, but, conversely may not mind skipping a day here or there because they are so consistent. Ultimately, it is about what value they are bringing to the table. Are they helping you or holding you back? I like to lift alone so that I don't have to adhere to someone else's schedule. But, I do a good job of motivating myself and find that I can easily blame a lazy partner for my absence in the gym.

Should I Take Creatine?
When I first tried to put weight on, Creatine had weird effects on me, but it might not for you. Many of my friends and people I look up to take it with fantastic results. I found that when I was skinnier, it would help me push through workouts and give me a great swell, for about two weeks, and then I would start to lose everything. Now I take it for brief periods with good results.

Should I Take a Pre-Workout?
 I'd say yes if you feel like you need the energy. I haven't had one yet that didn't give me a boost, but I have had a few that upset my stomach. If you feel like you have enough energy at the gym, I recommend limiting your intake of as much unregulated processed garbage as you can.

Gym Etiquette
Asking for help is perfectly acceptable if you're not stopping somebody mid-lift or bothering a trainer who is working with a client. Always stack your weights back on the rack and put them in the right order, even if you found them a mess. Do your part to help and take pride in the dojo where you will build your body. Don't yell like a madman. Wear shorts that will cover some of your legs at the very least. Don't creep on people. Clean off the machines after you've sweat all over them. Dropping weights is fine, but don't slam them. If there's a mirror on the wall, don't lean on it. If the gym is crowded, don't hog more than one station. Sharing is caring. Your water bottle, phone or whatever doesn't need its own bench. And always remember where you started (don't be a douche).

How I Gained 30lbs in Six Months While Maintaining Abs

I've broken down the lifestyle that I had during these six months in the beginning of this book, so I will avoid repeating those (extremely important) details for the sake of my readers with short attention spans (guilty). Keeping in mind that I just started stomach expansion at the beginning of this workout routine, so it took me well over a month to start seeing numbers on the scale. Once the diet reached a certain point, the flood gates were opened. At the time, I had a heavy focus on bench press thanks to some insecurities of mine and a chest-obsessed partner. We spent a good two hours on each session. The routine is listed below.

Mon: Chest/Shoulders/Triceps
Tues: Back/Biceps/Cardio/Core
Wed: Chest/Shoulders/Triceps
Thurs: Back/Biceps/Cardio/Core
Fri: Chest/Shoulders/Triceps

I wouldn't recommend this routine to anybody today. Unless you're in your early 20's or younger, it doesn't leave enough time to recoup. This routine focuses too much on 'glory muscles', and nowhere near enough on the important building blocks of bodybuilding. However, my early routine did have a few good things going for it. My max on bench was 185lbs when I started and it grew to 250lbs. But if you aren't competing, know that focusing on one muscle group like this is an incredibly inefficient way of building the overall body you want. I messed up my shoulder and elbow pretty bad by doing this. Putting too much focus on a specific muscle group can screw up your joints or even hurt your posture. I squatted every day. I saw significant improvements in the strength of those glory muscles. I packed on a ton of weight. And I had a lot of fun doing it.

A few other things to mention: On many of my cardio days, I was running upwards of 7mi, which really helped keep the fat off, but may have worked against my weight gain a bit. I was only 19 which allowed me to bounce back to the gym every day. Don't ignore the way I ate and the sleep I made sure to get. I also wasn't solely focused one weight gain. Rather, I was focused on strength.

Squat Every Day.
If legs are something you're not used to working, your squat max is looking a little light, you want to charge up your testosterone and improve all your lifts, lift legs frequently. If you want to get better at a specific skill (squats in this instance), put a focus on that skill. Before starting my routine listed above, I would religiously do 4 sets of squats at 8-10 reps per set. Squatting is well-known for increasing testosterone and helping build muscle everywhere. If you ignore your legs, you're doing yourself (and your intimate partner) a disservice. Squatting every day or even every other day is a game changer. Although you probably won't get sore after the first few days, it will make you stronger everywhere and should make you happier from the increased testosterone.

Other Tried-and-True Muscle Builders?
Other than squats, people swear by the deadlift and bench-press as the best overall muscle building exercises because of how they stimulate your body. I focus more on incline bench because of my build and believe more that the bigger muscles help you gain more mass. I also believe that dips and pull-ups work wonders for your shape, arm size, and help improve overall strength. If you can't do these, don't be embarrassed to use the assist or have a spotter. With a little practice, you will get much better. Try doing them first thing every day. Bottom line: don't neglect the tried and true, but also try the other routines I've mentioned. Do it all and build a balanced body. Below is a list of some of my favorites.

Table 1: List of Some Exercises I Perform Regularly (do a quick Google or Bodybuilding search for descriptions)**:**

Abs/Core	Triceps	Biceps
P90X Ab-Ripper X routine Kneeling Cable Crunch Hanging Leg Lifts Decline Weighted Sit-Ups Wood Choppers with Cables Spell Casters Dumbbell vs Land-mines One Arm Side Dead Lifts Lower Back Press Machine Deadlifts	Incline Bench Skull Crushers Extensions with Cables Overhead Dumbbell Press Body Weight Skull Crusher Skull Crusher Dumbbell Side Cable Extensions (at shoulder level) Kick Backs Reverse Grip Bench Press Dips	Incline Curls Rope Hammer Curls E-Z Bar Curls Preacher Curls (Dumbbell/Barbell) Standing Barbell Curl Standing Rows Chin-Ups Pull-Ups Reverse Grip Curls Romanian Curls Burnouts: Crazy-8's/21's
Chest	**Legs**	**Back**
Incline Dumbbell Press Flat Dumbbell Press Chest Machine Variants Flies Variants (Incline vs. Flat) Decline Barbell	Squat Variation (Front Squat vs Traditional) Romanian Deadlift Bulgarian Split Squat Leg Press Curls Squat Machine or Smith Machine	Reverse Grip Lat Pull-Downs/Traditional Grip Cable Rows Close/Wide Grip Machine Variants of above exercises Bent-Over Rows (Barbell/Dumbbell) Rear Flies Bent-Over Flies Back Extension

Press Decline Dumbbell Press Push-Ups Negatives	Single Leg Squats

Calves	**Shoulders and Traps**
Seated Calf Raises Standing Calf Raises Single Leg Press Stair Climber on Tiptoes	Military Press (Dumbbell/Barbell) Arnold Dumbbell Military Press with Shoulder Flies Single Arm Landmine Land Mine Shoulder-to-Shoulder Press Dumbbell Shoulder-to-Shoulder Press Bent-Over Rear Deltoid Fly (hands in neutral) High Incline Front-Facing Shoulder Press Leaning Lateral Raises Combo w/ other single joint moves Straight Arm Cable Kick-Back

Want Bigger Arms?

Focused approach. Try doing my favorite arm building exercises regularly: pull-ups and dips. Do these every day before you start the routine. If you lift chest and triceps together, start your routine focusing on triceps and end with chest. If your arms aren't sore, insert and arm day in between your other workouts. Keep in mind that triceps make up the bulk of your arms, so make sure you aren't neglecting these in anyway.

Want Bigger Forearms?

Build a roller by screwing a belt to the middle of cylinder of wood (think broom handle). Tie weight to the end of the belt. Roll the weight up and then slowly back down. You can do this for a few dollars. Do some research on how to put one of these together. Buy a grip strengthener. Squeezing objects that are big for your hands is better than objects that feel small. Bring a towel to the gym and wrap it around a bar for curls to increase the width. Wrap a towel around the pull-up bar on each side and hang onto the towel to focus on your grip.

Minimalist Approach: How I Gained 10lbs of Muscle in One Month

The opposite end of the spectrum can deliver incredible results as well. Instead of putting ten hours a week into the gym, try just putting in one! I read *The Four-Hour Body* by Tim Ferriss and was astonished at what this 'body hack' could deliver. Essentially, it comes down to a specialized routine that is laser focuses at shocking your muscles, and it is both extremely challenging and rewarding. I will attempt to break down the basics of how I interpreted it. Pick 8-10 multi-joint (i.e. elbow and shoulder in a bench press) exercises that encompass all muscle groups in the body (see my routine below). The book recommends coming up with two sets of these workouts and then alternating the routines in an A-day and B-day fashion. In only about a half an hour, attempt to complete **only one set** of each exercise with no more than eight total reps per exercise. The weight you use should be around 60% of your max. The catch: do each rep as slowly as you physically can. It is recommended to take 5 seconds on the way down, and 5 seconds up, but I found that I could go much slower on lifts for the core and legs. The first rep will make you laugh and question the validity of this routine. The last 2-3 reps will make you cry as if someone is poking the muscle you're working on with a hot iron while talking about your old childhood dog who had to be put down. **You should fail by 8 reps**. If you don't fail, slow down or increase the weight. See my example for day A:

Incline Bench Press with Dumbbells: 50lbs x 7 reps
Leg Press: 300lbs x 7 reps
Reverse Slide Curls: 40lbs x 8.5 reps (had to put down that extra half rep here)
Seated Calf Raises: 90lbs x 7 reps
Shoulder Press Machine: 118lbs x 6.5 reps
Supinated Close Grip Lat Pull-Downs: 80lbs x 7 reps
Weighted Dips: 25lbs x 4 reps
Leg Curls: 100lbs x 5 reps
Machine Crunch: 100lbs x 8reps
Deadlift: 135lbs x 7 reps

The craziest part is that you only need to work out two days a week to stay consistently sore. After committing to this routine for a month, I gained muscle and strength and even lost fat. I especially felt like it worked muscles and strengthened ligaments that I wasn't used to targeting. I want to mention that I was practicing the slow-carb diet at the time, which allowed me to eat copious amounts of protein and effectively cut fat. Had I not been dieting, I am sure I would've gained more. This is a great workout, one that I will come back to whenever I hit a wall. I would especially recommend considering this if you feel like you have absolutely no time to work out. The downsides to this routine are important to mention, but are not important in my opinion. For starters, you will look absolutely ridiculous doing this in public. Your arms will shake, you will make a face like you're pooping glass, you won't be lifting very heavy weight, and after gasping for air briefly following your two minutes of exercise, you will move onto another agonizing display in a different part of the gym. Like I said, none of this should matter to you if it works. The positive to these awkward side-effects: this routine is a great way to desensitize yourself from what others think about you.

My measurements after 4-Hour Body and Slow-Carb Diet for a Month:
December 5th to January 2nd Measurements:
Neck:16.75" to 17.25"
Right Bicep:15.25" to 16"
Shoulders:46.75" to 47.75"
Chest:41.75" to 42.75"
Right thigh:23" to 23.5"
Right calve:15" to 16"

Weight: 172lbs to182.5lbs

My Take on The Slow-Carb Diet:
Cut out all breads, starchy vegetables, and limit sugars (including fruits). Maximize your protein and fiber intake while considering stomach expansion for every meal. I ate 1.5g of protein minimum per pound of body weight which you can see below in a typical day.
Breakfast: Protein Shake, 2 eggs, yogurt, handful of spinach = ~50g protein
Snack: Beef Jerky (x5), Cashews = 40g protein
Lunch: Chicken Breast, Cheese Stick, Black Beans/Lentils = 80g protein
Snack: Protein Bar = 20g protein
Dinner: Chicken (x2)or equivalent source, Quinoa/Lentils/Black Beans, Kale = 80g protein
Snack: Casein Shake, Munchies = 30g protein

Remember to look at working out through a fresh lens. Imagine that you are going to the gym for the first time. Imagine that this is a new kind of gym designed to provide you with all the tools you need to bulk up. Constantly remind yourself of your mission. You will need to work hard to gain weight. You are fully capable of working hard and bulking up. Remind yourself while you're pushing out that last rep, and see if you can get one more. Remind yourself before you stack the weights that you are here to push yourself, and see if you can add a little more. Remember that you have a clear goal. You are already at the gym, so don't walk out until you know you gave it your everything!

I have attached a few example routines for pushing yourself and gaining weight. Feel free to interchange these with similar exercises or tweak them to your liking. Feel free to work out however you please and ignore my routines. Just be sure to push yourself and end on a good note!

Workout Plan Example 1: <u>Muscle Groups</u> Estimated Gym Time: 1.5-2hrs per session, 4 days on, 1-2 days off

Legs Core	1-2 of these exercises: Squats, Deadlifts, Leg-press; Leg Extensions; (1-2 of these) Lunges, Leg Curls, Kick-Backs; Calve Raises 3-4: Ab/Core exercises; Lower back crunch
Chest Triceps	3-4: Major Exercises with 1: Fly Variant to Burnout 2-3: Major Exercises with 1: Light-weight Burnout
Back Biceps/Forearms	3-4: Major Exercises with 1: Fly Variant to Burnout 2-3: Major Exercises with 1: Burnout / Curls, wrist twists dumbbells
Shoulders Trapezius	2-3: Major Exercises with 2: Fly Variants 1-2: High Set Shrug Variants (5+ sets)

Workout Plan Example 2: <u>Dividing Up the Week</u>: Estimated Gym Time 0.5-1hr per session, 5 days on, 1 day off. This plan could be stretched to divide biceps and triceps up into their own day. The shorter your gym session, the harder the gain. But anything is better than nothing, so do what you can and push yourself!

Legs	2-3: Major Exercises; 2-3: Lunges, Leg Curls, Kick-Backs; Calve Raises

Chest/ Abs	3-4: Major Exercises with 1: Fly Variant to Burnout 3-4: Ab Exercises sure to hit full range
Back/ Lower Back	3-4: Major Exercises with 1: Fly Variant to Burnout 2: Lower Back Crunch Variants
Tris/Bis	Super-Set: 2-3: Major Exercises with 1: Light-weight Burnout for each
Shoulders/ Trapezius	2-3: Major Exercises with 2: Fly Variants 1: Shrug Variant (4+ sets)

Workout Plan Example 3: Opposing Muscle Groups: Estimated gym time: 1-2hrs, 4 days on, 1-2 days off. *This can be done faster by easily super-setting.*

Legs Shoulders/Trapezius	2-3: Major Exercises with 2-3: Lunges, Leg Curls, Kick-Backs; Calve 1-2: High Set Shrug Variant (5+ sets)
Chest/ Back	3-4: Major Exercises with 1: Fly Variant to Burnout each
Biceps/ Triceps	3-4: Major Exercises with 1: Light-weight Burnout for each
Core	3-4: Ab/Core exercises; Lower back crunch (5+ sets)

Workout Plan Example 4: Opposing Muscle Groups #2:
Estimated gym time: 1-2hrs, 4 days on, 1-2 days off. *This can be done faster by easily super-setting.*

Legs/ Core	3-4: Lower back crunch 2-3: Lunges, Leg Curls, Kick-Backs; Calve 3-4: Ab/Core exercises; Lower Back Crunch (5+ sets)
Chest/ Biceps/Forearms	3-4: Major Exercises with 1: Fly Variant to Burnout for each
Back/ Triceps	3-4: Major Exercises with 1: Fly Variant to Burnout for each
Shoulder/ Traps	2-3: Major Exercises with 2: Fly Variants 1: Shrug Variant (4+ sets)

SLEEP

"I haven't slept for ten days... because that would just be too long." -Mitch Hedberg

There will be no gains without good sleep, so make sure you're balancing your life. If you work hard to build your body, make sure you are resting hard as well. You can't go out drinking every night and expect to build your ideal body. You probably shouldn't even go to the gym if you didn't sleep well the night before. On the other hand, if you haven't slept well for a while, working up a good sweat might help get you to sleep. My sleeping issues often come from not exercising or pushing myself enough. I find that when I really push myself, sleep is easy. Sleep is very beneficial for your physique, mood, and overall health. If you have the time, take a nap after the gym and prepare for amazement. If you're struggling with sleep, I've been there as well. Below are some of my sleep tips.

Diet:
Make sure you're sleeping on a full belly and that you've drank enough water throughout the day. If I'm not waking up to pee, I'm waking up because I'm uncomfortable from being dehydrated. Because Casein protein is slow digesting, it helps keep your belly full while you sleep. Avoid caffeine late at night. If I drink coffee past 3pm, I'll be awake half the night. If you are still feeling the effects of caffeine, try to burn some energy!

Sleep Aids:
I've tried so many. Lavender tea works wonders and tastes decently. Melatonin and valerian root work well. Word to the wise, valerian root smells awful. Other supplements like magnesium and potassium help many people sleep.

Earplugs:
Maybe you're a light sleeper like me. Getting used to wearing earplugs can really improve your sleep. I use a humidifier that also

provides some nice white noise. There are great white noise apps, websites and machines available.

CPAP:
If it seems like no matter how long you sleep you never feel awake during the day, try taking a sleep study. I'm not a big guy at all but apnea runs in the family and sure enough, I'd suffered 29 years with it progressively getting worse.

Stretch:
Stretch every day. Try some yoga. The more you work out, the tighter your body will get. I really can't stress the importance of stretching enough. I make it the first thing I do every day so I can be sure I'll do it. I also stretch before I get in bed, and my bed always feels more comfortable because of it.

Closing Thoughts

"Absorb what is useful, discard what is not, and add what is uniquely your own" -Bruce Lee

As you've read, I've experimented with many routines and I continue to experiment. Lifting and eating were extremely difficult habits to start, but I now find myself longing to go to the gym and find it difficult to eat less! This is me, a guy that has vivid memories of crying because he had to eat broccoli, could never clear his plate and wouldn't even finish a sandwich. If I can adapt, so can you. I enjoy testing the limits of my body. Once you realize you can break through these barriers that have held you back for so long, the sky is the limit. Stay committed. Stay positive. Stay Honest. You too will succeed. If you are looking for more advice, would like to share your thoughts (good and bad), I'm making myself available through email, Quora, and I just started blog. Feel free to reach out!

authorkhail@gmail.com

http://khail.space

www.ingramcontent.com/pod-product-compliance
Lightning Source LLC
Chambersburg PA
CBHW032032290526
45786CB00012B/2659